I0705635

Dedication

As a personal reverence and gratitude to my loving family, I dedicate this book to my mom who has worked very hard to raise us by compromising her career for the family. She has a double master's degree in Economics and Sociology from Miranda House College, New Delhi. I am sure she got success in raising all her kids with good values. On the other hand, my father who was a doctor did tremendous work in helping everyone who needed him. All our family members have been the direct beneficiaries of my father's presence, guidance, financial and moral support during his entire lifespan. He had a great sense of discipline, yet so loving, and created a bonding among the entire family.

We in our humble ways remember him so affectionately for our upbringing and make no distinctions among the family members.

He gave the entire family the best academic education, high moral values which helped us in building good character in life. These virtues were so dear to him.

I dedicate this book to my parent's memory so that it inspires the readers to imbibe some of their rare qualities which would always help them in facing the challenges of life.

Acknowledgement

Writing a book is harder than I thought and more rewarding than I could have ever imagined. None of this would have been possible without my Husband, Mr. Ratan Bajpai. He is my best friend. He stood by me during my every struggle and all my life's success.

I'm eternally grateful to my uncle Mr. Padmakar Shukla, who has been my role model during my entire life and became a father figure after my father's death. Also, my aunt Mrs. Prabha Shukla (RIP) gave me love and care to become successful in life.

I want to thank my uncle Dr. Ashok Goyal for his care, love, support, and hospitality for the last twenty-two years.

Sincere gratitude to my family: my kids Rohan and Eshaan, Uncle Mr. Shanti. P. Dwivedi (Retd Principal of N.M.D college, Gondia, India) and to all Dwivedi family, father-in-law Mr. Narendra Bajpai, mother-in-law Mrs. Kusum Bajpai and to all Bajpai family. Thank you for letting me know that you have nothing but great memories of me. So thankful to have you in my life.

To my babysitter (RIP) Mrs. Kashi Bai Baune (Bai): for the social and emotional support, she gave me in the early development of my life, This had a great impact throughout my life to shape me with confidence, to meeting new people, and overcoming difficult situations. I will always have a soft feeling for her the way she raised me. I never knew that I needed her support and that it will help me for years to come.

Finally, Thanks to Saraswati Vidyalaya Nagpur, Hadas High School, Nagpur, Sevagram Engineering College (BDCOE), Wardha, and Indian Institute of Management Development, Nagpur for providing me the education to help me reach where I am today.

Preface

This preface attempts to answer the question, "Why should I read this book?"

People around the world regardless of race, gender, education, rich or poor do not think about how they can improve their lives by making good decisions. Quite a few people are in a rat race by copying others and living an unhappy life. They regret their lives later. Blaming others for our mistakes doesn't help. We all need self-improvement and re-investing in ourselves (by accepting our mistakes and correcting them) every few years to live better. Many times, common sense is uncommon in common people.

With my 29 years of Meditation and 20 years, both as an Engineering and M.B.A experience in IT, I think life is an examination and it is a mixture of failure and success. For me, failure comes first then success. I have tried different methods and learned how to overcome hard situations in a smart way. How to manage time and energy in an effective way to live a better life.

We live in the internet age and have vast amounts of information floating everywhere. It's hard to find good information in this vast universe. It's like looking for good gems in a vast ocean of knowledge. Maybe you can find some better knowledge on the internet but not all in one book. I have collected some of my good and bad experiences on how to live a better life. Meditation is the best technique to control your mind and body. With a healthy mind and body, you can make better decisions. We are lacking knowledge and are confused in life about what to do next. This book is a guide that you can implement after reading. It has a few important tips or secrets. It all depends on how to interpret it. Humans around the world have similar types of mindsets and no guidance to move forward in life. I'm hoping after reading this book you will be able to make good decisions to live your life better.

Contents

It's My Life

What is Life? Sometimes it is hard to understand it. Life is beautiful! It all depends on how you want to turn your life by making the right decision at the right time. Sometimes you have to live with those decisions for the rest of your life. They may not be what you always want. There are no shortcuts. Shortcuts are often wrong cuts. It is not as simple as playing video games where you just press the button and get the result. You have to practice every day to make it beautiful. Hard work and determination are needed to make your desires come true.

There are different stages in life as we grow and learn from them. We cannot change the whole world, so it is easy to change ourselves to live better. The sooner we understand this, the better it is to adjust with others in a balanced way. We can develop few good habits to optimize the time in our life. The journey of life starts when we are born. Infants are innocent and bold to do the right things that they like. We as parents change them so that they can survive in this world. Sometimes parents make the right decision when trying to change the habits of their kids, whereas at other times they do not. Only a few habits can be changed when kids are young, when they grow old, they keep pushing and do things their own way. Everyone has some natural talents; it all depends upon how they want to use their talents to get better results. I have written a few experiences of my life to illustrate how I have changed myself to live a better life.

When I was seven months old my mom got typhoid. She had to take the help of a babysitter to raise me. I started sleeping with my babysitter as I was scared at night and didn't want to sleep in my little bed. I was emotionally attached to my babysitter. I think she was in her sixties at that time. I used to call her Bai. She was a good woman, and people used to think that she was my grandma. I used to share all my secrets with her. When she used to take a vacation, it was so hard to live without her for a few days. I used to go to the bus stop every day to see if she is back. When she was back, that used to be the happiest day of my life. Babysitter and kids sometimes develop deep bonds between themselves which may never be forgotten.

At the age of three or four, we as kids start forming memories. I still remember the childhood time I had spent with my dad. I was my daddy's girl. When I was three and half years old, every morning after getting up, I used to sing some rhymes with my dad. He was a doctor and used to come late at night from his clinic. By the time he was home, I used to be in bed already. The morning was good for us to spend time together with lots of fun. Over the weekends we used to clean our fish tank and I used to help him by singing a song for the fishes so that the fishes can live longer.

When I was in pre-k, I didn't like to go to school and used to make a lot of excuses. My dad used to trick me by telling me that we are going to a toy shop and used to drop me at school. I think every day was the same story. One day my dad asked me why I didn't want to go to school. My school was in a small town, and all the kids used to sit on the rug for 2 or 3 hours. I told my dad that I didn't like sitting on the floor as it hurts my legs. Also, I told him that I should get some good candies during the lunch break. He talked to my teacher and the teacher agreed that I will sit on a chair. The teacher used to sit on one side whereas I was on the other side of the classroom. All the other kids used to sit on the floor. With these changes, it became easy for me to attend pre-k. I got VIP treatment due to my dad, and the teachers did not teach me much. This pattern continued for a few years.

My dad was the highest-paid doctor in the town as he was professionally very good. Most people knew about him. He helped everyone and many poor people in the town who didn't have money for their treatment. In return, some patients like the vegetable sellers, used to bring fresh vegetables for my dad. He tried not to take those as they can get money after selling the vegetables. He was a kind and well-known doctor in the town. After spending few years in small towns my dad was forced to take a transfer to the city as my mom didn't want to live in a small town. She was from New Delhi. My dad finally transferred to Nagpur city. There he joined the Leprosy department. At that time due to lack of knowledge people used to treat leprosy patients badly as they had a fear of contracting the disease from them. My dad treated a lot of patients and did his research and told everyone that leprosy was not contagious.

After moving to the city, I got admission directly to the second grade by skipping KG and first grade. My older sister got in third grade. My sister came up to the speed by working hard during the summer vacation. Whereas I was more focused on playing with dolls and running around. My life was different from my sister's. We both are opposite personalities. She did well in school. But for myself, it was hard to memorize everything in my brain as it took a long time and I didn't want to cut the hours of my playtime. My life was different as I was living in my playful world. I was a happy and smart kid, but I was not focused on my studies and was playing all day. I think grades are just numbers in your mark sheet to make you feel good about yourself. It does not matter how you performed in school. Life is long and it will give you other opportunities to prove yourself. If there is a will, then there is a way to do better at any point in your life.

During summer vacation we used to go to our grandparent's town every year for two months. We used to play board games with our uncles for hours. Once my mom and uncles started giving us tips for the morning routine. They insisted us to develop a morning routine. It was hard as a kid to follow the routine but later it become our habit. Our aunts with the help of helpers worked hard to cook good food for all of us during the hot summer months. We did a few road trips with our extended families. We developed strong bonds with our aunts as we spent a lot of time with them talking about different topics. Sometimes parents push their kids hard to learn good habits when they are young, which later helps them throughout their life.

We had a baby brother come into our life when I was in fifth grade. I was so focused on playing that I didn't know that my mom was pregnant till she started going to the doctor. I was worried all time about my mom's health as I didn't want to lose her. My Aunt came to help us during that time. She used to tell us a story every night before going to bed. Those stories with good lessons are stuck in my brain forever. Storytelling is good for kids. I think that helped me to grow and understand how humans think and act in different situations.

I started skipping school for few days as I was excited to spend time with my baby brother at home. After missing school for a few days, my teacher noticed and asked me about being absent from school. She got upset about this. One day before school started, she punished me by slapping me. It was a shameful experience in front of other students. It hurt pretty bad both physically and emotionally. I cried for some time. I went home and did not share this with my mom. I was afraid that she will come to school to talk to the teacher and the teacher will retaliate. This happened in the third grade too. My teachers made some hard decisions regarding me missing the studies, and that hurt my feelings pretty badly. After that, I started focusing on my studies from sixth grade onwards. My older sister was my role model as she was academically very good. I followed her schedule. She used to study a lot to get good grades. I was confused with our school's teaching method as we had to memorize everything instead of developing an understanding. It was hard for me and for that reason I only understood math well. It was easy to understand what is going on after seeing the results. I developed a lot of interest in math as compared to other subjects. I didn't like history as I was not interested in knowing what happened in the past.

During my school years in India, teachers were mean to the students who were not strong academically. I went through this grueling process for years. There is another incident from sixth grade that I remember vividly. During that grade, my teachers pushed me hard to change my handwriting from straight to cursive. I somehow changed it, but my overall handwriting became pretty bad after that. My teachers were upset with my new handwriting for years until I finished high school. In my school, sometimes teachers pushed the students pretty hard, so instead of learning a better habit, kids just remembered the mean things teachers did. I still think they were my gurus and I should respect them. My tough experiences helped me to become a stronger person. I have done a lot better in life than my teachers expected me to do.

When I was a kid, we used to go to Ramakrishna Mission with my dad. One of the reasons my dad used to go to Ramakrishna Mission was that his cousin become a saint there. The other reason was that my dad wanted to do volunteer work to help others as a doctor. My uncle was a math gold medalist who joined Ramakrishna Mission to become a saint. After a few years, he become the general secretary of the mission at Calcutta. Going to Ramakrishna Mission felt good to me because I could skip my studies. I didn't have any interest in learning religious prayers. My only motivation was that we will get some sweets as prasad to eat after the prayer. I heard a lot of good stories about Swami Vivekananda there. Those teachings, stories, and good values lasted with me throughout my life. I think we did this for a few years until went to high school. I believe going to Ramakrishna Mission helped me in many ways to adopt good behavior and values.

My mom played a bigger role in changing my life by pushing me hard. She had great discipline at home, and we all had to follow it without any excuse. She used to give us several good examples so that we can become good kids. One of the examples was that the owl is the wisest animal as it listens more and talks less. She used to say follow the owl's qualities to become wise. I thought she was right as we should speak less and listen more, and I tried to follow her advice. She was a protective mom. I used to get upset when we were not allowed to go out in the dark to play. But now I realize that she did the right thing as a mom.

I remember when I was in middle school, we used to like watching TV for hours whether it was of interest or not. At that time, we used to have limited channels. My mom used to tell us every day that we were wasting our time watching bad TV shows instead of focusing on our studies. At that age, I didn't like her advice. But later on, due to the pressure of my studies in high school, I stopped watching TV. I had to push myself hard during that time on not watching TV. Later it become my habit and I lost interest in watching TV. I am not a TV person and will use my time in doing some other work of my interest. All the hard work and good discipline of my mom forced us to develop good habits and lead a better life.

Soon after graduating from high school, I was in a dilemma on which career to pursue. I was from a family of doctors and lawyers. In high school, I took both biology and math. I was having a hard time deciding what field to pursue. My mom suggested me to become a doctor. I was passionate about math and wanted to pursue that to become an engineer. My dad suggested if I want, I can take civil engineering as a major because it was a hot field in his time. In the 90s, girls were more interested in electronics engineering as compared to civil engineering. I finally got admission in electronics engineering but did not get the school of my choice and had to go to another school. It was not a bad school and had similar fee, but my attitude was not good about it, to begin with. If you start something new with a bad attitude, you are more likely to experience bad things. Attitude matters in life. If I can go back in the past and change my decision, I would have liked to become an interior designer or maybe a doctor. I don't have many regrets but kids at that age are mostly confused and it's better to listen to your parents as they also went through the same stage in their life.

When I was in engineering school, a life-changing event happened to me when my younger sister died in an accident. That changed my whole life. It hurt so bad at that time. You don't have any control over the life and death of someone that you love the most. She was my best friend. No one can replace her spot in my heart and it still feels like life is hollow without her. It impacted my personality in many ways. I remember some people came over for expressing their condolences. The way they expressed their feelings by using the wrong choice of words made it very insensitive. Some people are insensitive to other people's feelings as they did not go through the same pain in their life. The unfortunate truth is that people will always remember bad words more than the good things that you did to them. But life is life and we all have to live with it. You have to change yourself, ignore the negative experiences, and move forward.

After graduating I joined my first job and was happy with it. My job was in the MIDC industrial area, but I did not continue there for long. The commute to work was fifteen kilometers from my home. It was hard to drive a two-wheeler which was not in a good condition. There was always some problem when it rained. The two-wheeler would stop working. Because of all these troubles, I left the job after working there for a few months. The good part about Indian parents is that they pay for all your college fees and you can stay with them after graduation until you get a job. I was staying at home with my parents without a job for a few years. Life was awesome with friends as no responsibilities and a lot of freedom.

My family started asking me to get married. I can either find someone myself or they can look for an arranged marriage. My parents were very open-minded. My mom always used to suggest that if you love someone then you should marry that person as life is a long way to go. She thought it is easier to adjust in love rather than arranged marriage. I agreed with my mom, but I was not able to find a suitable person. I decided to go with arranged marriage. I had made a checklist to find a husband. My criteria for marriage were different as I used to think that I just didn't want to marry any boy. The family is important too. For a long-lasting relationship, the boy should be from a good family like mine. Education was important to me, so I was looking for someone with a master's degree. I was very picky about everything in life. My concept was to get married only once in life. I didn't want to repeat the same mistake again if my marriage did not work. I know a few people rush to marry and then are unsuccessful in their marriage. I know checklist for a husband sounds weird. Luckily a few boys were able to match my criteria, and I decided to marry one of them after meeting him a few times. We went to Paris for our honeymoon and then came to the US.

I had never done any home chores in India before marriage. My mom used to say we should learn good qualities on how to keep our home clean and organized. After coming to the US I started doing cooking and other chores. My parents taught me a few good tips to adjust in life as no marriage is perfect. I listened to them and followed their advice. I joined my first job in the US in a telecommunications company. Marriage is a lot of hard work and adjustment. Both partners have to work together to make it successful. I also had ups and downs in the initial adjustment phase of married life. Soon after my marriage, my dad passed away. It hit me hard again with no choice other than to live my life with pain. It took months and years to overcome this type of heartbroken feeling.

We planned two kids and are lucky to have them in our life. To have a baby is the most wonderful experience in the world. For some reason, both of my pregnancies were hard as I had gestational diabetes. I used to take insulin three times a day and blood tests six times a day for the last 10 weeks of both pregnancies. After looking at my baby's face, I didn't remember any of those pains. Both boys were delivered healthy, and that mattered the most.

It is never easy to raise kids when you are a working woman. With minimum extended family support, it was very challenging to raise the boys. But somehow, we finally managed it. I feel I could have done better when raising my first son as compared to the little one. It was sometimes hard to find accurate information on the internet regarding raising infants. Being first-time parents, we did make mistakes along the way. We learned from those and did a better job the second time around. I am lucky to be their mom. They are both smart kids. I have learned a lot of things from them. They make me laugh for hours and care for me the most. I hope they will learn some good values from us to become good citizens.

Although life gets pretty hectic with both of us working, we try to balance out by taking time off to visit family and friends. My husband works hard for our family, speaks to our kids gently, and treats me with respect. He is a good husband. I also work hard for our family, treat his family and friends well, treat him well as he is the only man in my life. We both have a good sense of humor and we laugh together more often enjoying each other's company. We treat each other with kindness and respect. We are still in love, and happy in our relationship, and that matters the most.

From this point on, I'm wondering how the future course will be in our lives, and what to expect. Some people have talked about the mid-life crisis in their 40s. I think it is not related to gender or race or income. People feel unhappy and may hit their lowest point in life. If you're a parent with school-going kids, you have to work like a machine from morning till night without a break for several years. This can result in a burnout. Sometimes parents may be experiencing this unhappiness due to financial hardships. I think we have to stay focused and take necessary breaks to keep re-charging ourselves periodically. Also, we should make smart decisions for our financial health as discussed in the later part of this book.

After the kids are settled, most of the responsibilities are taken care of. Some people become financially independent by that time. They enjoy with their partner, friends, and grandkids. As we grow older, we see changes in ourselves. We try to live life the way we are and focus on the right things. By that time, we have the wisdom and experience to see what matters in life. Golden years are normally full of content and happiness if your health is good.

Summary:

- As humans, we get attached to people with whom we have spent a lot of time. They do not need to be related to us.

- Love your kids the way they are, don't force them to become perfect kids. Some habits you can change when they are young. Putting them in a lot of classes doesn't help. Instead of that try to spend more time with them to develop strong bonds. Childhood memories stay with kids throughout their life, so they should be pleasant. Strictness doesn't help as kids start hiding the truth from their parents. Be open-minded to have discussions with them. Kids learn their core values at home by watching their parent's behavior all the time.

- Tell your kids any good stories at home as stories are sticky. They remember stories all their lives and learn good lessons from them. If possible, tell them some religious stories but focus on spirituality. This may help them not to pick bad habits of drinking and smoking during their teenage. It is very hard to get rid of these addictions.

- Listen to your parents especially when making career decisions as they have more knowledge and experience than you. Keep your ears open to listen to everyone's feedback but make your own decisions based on your feelings.

- Spend some time finding the right spouse for your marriage as it is full of compromise and adjustment. Also, plan your family carefully whenever you're ready to take up the responsibility.

- If you are married with kids and have disagreements with your spouse, try to rethink your relationship. Separation or divorce has a bad impact on kids. Kids suffer the most.

- Nobody knows better about yourself than you, so believe in yourself and think positive. Avoid listening to what other people say about you. Practice good habits by doing the things on time that can help you to lead a better life.

- Be true to yourself who you are. Don't try to please everyone by suppressing yourself. Don't pretend to be someone else when other people don't see your worth. Many people will come and go in your life, but the good ones will stay.

- Good attitude matters in life. Hard work and discipline are the keys to success. Don't be scared of failures. Sometimes failure is the first step to success. Don't remain in a failure state for long. Failure is not the end of the world, get up and fight again until you get success. Remember all the great leaders failed several times before becoming great.

- Avoid becoming a technology slave. Take some break with less screen time. Do outside exercise as it is more beneficial to your body than indoor exercise. Don't stay alone. Hang out with the people you like by going on lunch or dinner with them. Join some community or social group. Socialization and friendship are important for us to grow as we are all human beings.

Lastly, I believe whatever good we do to others is sometimes for our satisfaction so that we don't have regrets later in life. Other chapters in this book are also based on my experience about life but they are written in a way of a life coach to live a better life.

Meditation Benefits

Meditation is a technique to train your mind to see the good things and enjoy the present moment in life. It is the best way to relax your mind. We all live in a busy world. Our mind is always very busy processing something all the time except while sleeping. Do we ever get time to relax our mind without screen time or reading or cooking or playing or just doing nothing? Maybe some people will think it will be a waste of time. But your mind needs to get some break from this daily routine. For example, when we have pain in the neck or leg, we go to a doctor, but for our brain, we never think about it until we have serious mental problems. Our brain is like a CPU and always processing something throughout the day without break. Whatever good or bad input we feed to our brain, it processes and acts on it. So, we should be feeding the right information to our brains. Our brain is a machine that needs maintenance to live better.

Meditation is a natural way to give some mental relaxation to your brain that forces the brain to think positively about life and decreases negative thoughts about yourself. Meditation slows down the hyperactivity of the brain. It focuses your concentration and increases your attention span. In this way, you control your brain to do logical and rational thinking. Meditation helps to develop a deep connection for a meaningful life and cultivate self-awareness for the present moments by clearing your thoughts. You will get the answer to all your unsolved questions and will start relating with the people around you. It will boost your confidence and self-esteem. It helps you to become a better person in the long run. So, it is important to clear your thoughts, keep calm, and feel good about yourself.

Meditation has the beauty to change the presence of the mind to focus only on the present moment. Relax and recharge your mind by sitting calmly.

In short, meditation is the science for a meaningful life for happiness, compassion, kindness, love, empathy, inspiration, and gratitude.

I have been doing meditation since I was an engineering college student, but I was not having any knowledge about it. I remember after revising all the material for hours, I was so focused and intense that after closing my eyes I used to review all the content in my brain. It may be around 50 or 60 pages of the book, with remembering the exact page numbers too. It is a Visual Meditation technique that acts on the core of my brain. I still remember a lot of incidents that happened in my childhood with exact dates. It is good and bad sometimes if you remember everything. I used to have sleeping problems since childhood. After doing meditation I have improved my sleep. I have changed the focus of my meditation to some other things. I can predict a few future things. One of the examples is when I drive the car I can predict when another driver will be changing the lane. This has helped me avoid accidents a few times on the highway. Now I am an expert in doing meditation and can do it anytime, anywhere to relax myself. Meditation has given me the power to become a strong person to fight with life. I believe meditation is the best way to control your mind and body. It has a lot of benefits and some of them are mentioned below.

- **Memory Improvement**: Meditation helps you to sharpen your memory by concentrating and focusing on your goals. It changes your brain's signals for reasonable thinking. It is a mental exercise that acts on your brain and plays a key role to execute multiple cognitive tasks at a time.

- **Better Sleep**: If you have insomnia, then meditation helps to improve the quality of sleep. After lying down on the bed, if you do meditation, then it will relax your mind and body. You will fall asleep sooner and will stay asleep longer.

- **Pain Management**: It gives positive signals to your brain to cope up with the pain. It reduces pain sensations in the body and builds strength to overcome pain. Sometimes the pain is psychological rather than physical.

- **Addiction Recovery**: Meditation makes you emotionally stronger so that you can undergo treatment for your cravings and addictions. It gives you the internal strength to self-regulate and strengthen your willpower. It helps in your understanding to handle the situation better.

- **Reduces Depression**: We have to keep our brain busy by doing something otherwise: "An empty brain is a devil's workshop". Meditation changes your brain chemistry to focus on positive thinking. It also helps to overcome mood swings and sadness.

Practicing Meditation: Try different styles of meditation so that you can choose which one is good for you. If you want, you can find several styles on the internet. Meditation has different techniques about how to focus and control your mind to find internal peace. You can practice meditation anytime anywhere when you have 10 or 15 minutes during the day. Start with at least 10 minutes per day for a week to see the difference. If you can practice 30 minutes per day, then you will notice the difference quicker. You don't have to sit in a specific position and say 'OM' to do it. It will be better if you practice more, then you will become an expert in doing it anywhere, anytime. Close your eyes while doing meditation as eyes are the biggest distraction for your brain. Do meditation for a month without breaking it and you will enjoy doing it. You will see the benefits of it and will reach a stage where you have enhanced your performance. It will give you the ability to focus on your goals longer than others.

Some meditation techniques are below:

- **Body Scan Meditation:** Lay down or sit down and close your eyes. Start leading your awareness away from the brain to different parts of the body. First, start focusing mental attention on your feet and move up to your head while scanning for sensations, thoughts, and feelings. Screen all the body parts without judging them. When you reach your head focus on the center of your forehead for a few seconds and keep repeating it.

- **Visual Meditation:** Sit down and look at any statue-like Buddha for calming your mind. Close your eyes and guide your brain to create a mental image of that statue and pay attention to the sensations that arise.

- **Music Meditation:** Sit down, close your eyes and listen to calm music. Invite awareness while vibrations from the sound flow through the whole body. Focus on the sound, the present moment, and sensations created in the body. Sometimes people also dance while performing music meditation.

- **Focused Meditation:** It is like a breathing exercise. Close your eyes and start taking a slow deep breath in and out. Relax and focus your mind to observe the breath coming in and going out.

Summary: No one is perfect on this earth, but we can transform ourselves to live better. Focus on good things and ignore what we cannot change in life. We cannot change every little thing that happens the way we expect it. Meditation helps you to be more attentive to the present moment. It gives you awareness and a deep understanding of life. It helps you concentrate and focus on your goals to live a better life.

Healthy Lifestyle

Health is wealth! Health plays an important role in your life. If you are not healthy it is hard to live every day. If you are bedridden then it is a pain for both the patient and the caretaker. For good health, you need a stronger immune system, and for that, you have to work on your health for years. A healthy lifestyle to boost your immune system can be achieved by doing the following.

- Eat Healthy and Less

- Drink Water

- Do Regular Exercise

- Get Enough Sleep

- Avoid Alcohol and Smoking

- Vitamin Supplements

- Take Care of Yourself

- Reduce Stress

Eat Healthy and Less

When you eat unhealthy food like canned food, processed food, or packaged food with a lot of preservatives, your body will become unhealthy. Similarly, fatty and frozen foods are also not good for health. Your body will absorb the preservatives and other chemicals and it will increase the risk for obesity. The body mass index will go high, and it may weaken your immune system. You will be deprived of the antioxidants and nutrients needed to help grow your body stronger. This can later increase the chances of bad health and chronic diseases, such as diabetes, heart disease, and cancer.

Bad health can be avoided by eating freshly cooked vegetables with garlic, ginger, and turmeric that can boost the immune system. Instead of eating one big meal take small meals during the day. Do fasting in between meals for a few hours. A small intake of food will keep you in shape. Occasionally buffet is good but not every week. Intake of diet should be of fresh fruits, fresh vegetables, dairy, yogurt, nuts, seeds, legumes, whole grains, and some fresh meat like chicken or fish. Avoid frozen food and red meat as you never know how they process it and whether the animals have any diseases. Cut sugar and carbohydrates from your diet. The body breaks down or converts most carbohydrates into sugar or glucose. Sugar is sweet poison. A high intake of sugar causes inflammation in your body, and then this high inflammation takes your immune system down. Try a variety of food so that you can develop taste for different foods. Use different cooking oil every few months, it also helps to boost your immune system.

Drink Water

Drink one glass of water as you get up in the morning. It flushes all the good saliva you have in your mouth to your body and helps in boosting your immune system. Avoid sugary beverages as they are made of artificial flavors and have a lot of chemicals, which is not good for your health. Drink around six to eight glasses of water if you can, to keep you hydrated during the day. But if you drink too much water, then it will wash out all the good nutrients from your body.

Regular Exercise

My dad used to say that walking is the best exercise. Later we came to know that more scientific research was done on walking. Walking is one of the easiest and most effective forms of exercise. If you can walk 30 minutes every day outside, then you will see several benefits of how it can improve your health. Some of the benefits of walking are:

Boosts Immune System: Regular walking can help protect you from getting cold, flu, or other immune-related diseases.

Eases pain: In my personal experience walking also helps relieve pain from stiffness in your body as you forget the pain when you walk. It makes your body easier to move.

Reduces stress: Walking helps you feel relaxed in the fresh air. When you walk outside you come across other walkers and talk to them which changes your brain signals for a positive attitude as well as changes your mood swings.

- **Increases Energy Levels:** Walking increases blood flow in your body. The blood contains oxygen and nutrients which will be supplied to the muscles in the legs as well as the brain. This way you don't feel tired and it gives you energy.

- **Improves Overall Health:** Walking is a cardio exercise that reduces the risk of causing damage to your heart. It also helps in preventing diabetes, high blood pressure, and heart attack.

- **Extends Life Expectancy:** Walking has also been linked to decrease the risk of mortality, and a longer life expectancy.

Running is good and burns more calories but has a direct impact on your joints. For regular exercise, you need good joints. Biking is also good and safe with less stress on joints for those who are overweight or who have arthritis.

Regular exercise also leads to a better heart, lower sugar and blood pressure, reduces the risk of obesity, reduces the risk of chronic diseases, and increases metabolism. It is recommended to exercise around 150 minutes per week. Rest depends upon person to person.

Get Enough Sleep

Sleeping has a direct impact on your health. If you don't sleep well then, your brain will not function, and your body will not have the energy to perform all the activities. Everyone is different and has different sleep patterns. Some need eight hours of sleep and some need more than that. Children need ten to twelve hours of sleep. Understand your sleep requirements and act on them. Less sleep may lead to increased risk for chronic diseases and increased levels of stress hormones.

For having a good sleep unwind at least 30 minutes before bed and make your room dark with no electronic gadgets in your room. To form a regular sleeping pattern, sleep every day at the same time.

Avoid Smoking and Alcohol

Smoking and heavy drinking are very harmful to your health. There are no benefits of smoking as it damages the lungs. Excessive alcohol consumption leads to liver damage and will slowly start damaging your brain. Both will weaken your immune system.

Vitamin Supplements

We are not getting enough nutrients from our diet alone and for that reason, we need to consume some supplements, which help to boost the immune system such as Omega 3 fatty acids, Zinc, Magnesium, Vitamin B12, Vitamin D, and others. The fact about these vitamin supplements is that you never know how much your body will absorb them. Keep in mind sometimes supplements have side effects too. But if you are a poor eater then it is a good idea to take help from these vitamins. Try to get vitamins from natural sources like eating nuts, seeds, fresh fruits, and vegetables. You may get Vitamin D from the morning sunlight. Not enough Vitamin D can lead to cardiovascular disease, cancer, or early death.

Take Care of Yourself

For good health you have to take care of yourself, nobody else will. Don't miss your annual doctor's appointment as you will know all your blood test numbers. It also helps in detecting early illness if any.

Go for a dental cleaning at least once a year so that you will know the overall health of your teeth and gums. Limit cold water, ice cream, and sugar as they directly damage the teeth. Teeth play an important role in your health and keep your smile looking beautiful.

Get your eyes checked up every other year so that you know if they are in good condition.

Listen to your body or your inner voice. If you have any pain or anything bothering you, then take an immediate doctor's appointment so that you can catch the disease at an early stage. If you are suffering from flu symptoms, make sure to get enough rest. A quick snooze during the day and drinking a lot of fluids helps you recover from it faster.

Reduce Stress

Stress is the number one killer. Sometimes chronic stress may cause sleep disruption and make your brain hyperactive throughout the night. When we are under stress, our body releases hormones that are bad for our health. This can cause high blood pressure or heart attack. For chronic stress take immediate actions to reduce stress levels and allow your bodies to return to a normal state. Take the help of meditation to relax your brain.

Summary: Health is inside out. When you are healthy from the inside then you look good from the outside. There will be a glow on your face. Food is cheap, but health is expensive. Stay healthy so that you can enjoy a good life with fewer medical bills. For good health try to eat three fruits every day if possible: apple, banana, and orange.

Love & Relationship

Love is a true feeling for someone without judging them. It is never easy, never perfect, and always comes with disagreements and fights. We girls believe in fairytales. How can we get a perfect guy in this imperfect world where no one is perfect? We should keep our hopes lower to live a happy life as love is not a fairytale.

First love is like skydiving with fears, the more you fear, the less the chances of surviving at first love. It is the perfect chemistry between two people. Being more sensitive to your feelings just by doing what you feel good, without hoping for any rewards. Lovers feel more powerful as they are bonded to each other. First love is always unique, intense, and memorable that you never forget in life. You might be at a point in time where you will feel disconnected from the world as you are deeply involved in thinking about someone who feels exactly how you feel about them. It will boost and make you feel more confident about your views and beliefs. It's the physical and emotional intimacy of sharing all your secrets and uncomfortable thoughts that are not shared with anyone in life. It may shape who you are.

When you are in a new relationship, things around you seem a lot exciting. Sometimes chances are teens could neglect their studies and overlook their friends and family. Most people have more trust and openness in first love, which may later help to develop one's personality. First love in late teens or early twenties lasts longer as they are innocent at that age and flexible to adjust with each other with fewer expectations. These couples may end up marrying and living a happy life.

There is a difference between first love and love at first sight. Love, at first sight, happens fast and sometimes goes away fast too. Falling in love is easy but holding that for a long time is tough as you have to deal with realities. Every relationship has a honeymoon period. As soon it is over you have to land on earth to face the reality of each other.

Finding the right life partner is the biggest challenge unless you fall in love with someone. Normally people don't do much research in finding the right partner. They just go with the flow and later regret their decisions in life. It is better to take out some time from your busy routine and do some planning on what you are looking for in a partner. A wise man once said that before marrying a girl, look at her mother. Girls normally get the same genetic traits from their mother and will be the same way as their mother was. Women are like the root of the tree for a healthy family. They work hard under the ground so that the family tree can grow stronger and bear good fruits. We need only one good life partner to spend our whole life with. Once you find them, hold on to them for your dear life.

Most of the dating sites don't work in the end. You may find someone quicker on those sites but it will not last long. A long-lasting happy marriage is when you fall in love with your high school sweetheart or best friend and marry them. The reason behind this is that when you are young, you are more flexible to adjust and don't do all the calculations in life. You don't have past bad experiences in your relationship. All good relationships need adjustments and compromise. Age plays an important role in relationships. As we grow older, our choices are limited. We become rigid, hard to change our opinion, and go through bad experiences in relationships. At that point, we don't change the way we want to live our life.

Romeo and Juliet's love was famous because they did not marry. Otherwise, William Shakespeare would have written a different married couple story. Once you get married, life changes. Love is not what it seems like before. Everyone has to work hard to make their relationship successful. Luck has nothing to do with it. It is like when two imperfect individuals decide to make their relationship work long term. Marriage is compromise, respect, having patience, and forgiveness.

For a healthy relationship, the best way is to have face-to-face communication instead of calling or texting. Communication is the key and always reminds you of the things you love about your partner. The second is having regular sex depending upon each other's needs. If the love meter goes down, then the fight increases. The third is, to be honest with each other and discuss what is working and what is not working between couples. Fourth is to always support each other in public and correct each other in private. Fifth is to work hard and if possible, take more responsibility than your spouse. This will help him/her to make the relationship work with kindness and respect. Couples should share the load for household chores and should have a concept of one family and teamwork to help each other.

Every couple fights now and then, but the frequency of the fight matters. Couples have to find ways to remove their differences and stay healthy in the relationship. Sometimes they break one another's hearts and their marriage hangs on the thinnest threads. But through efforts, they can save their marriage as they don't want to lose each other. Marriage can be a very rewarding and enriching experience. It is important for a stable family unit.

A relationship is a two-way street. It affects you psychologically, physically, emotionally, mentally, and monetarily. It needs continuous efforts to maintain a relationship. You cannot just leave and neglect unsolved issues as it will create distances. It takes years to build a good relationship and no time to break it. Relationships are sensitive and delicate like glass. Once there is a small crack, it keeps growing until you try hard to fix it with patience and understanding.

Sometimes daily stress triggers unhealthy relationships. Due to good and bad days, we go through ups and downs now and then and get frustrated. However, it is normal until it becomes a trend, then it may be the sign of a bigger problem. How you manage disagreements and overcome them is important. If you cannot resolve your issues after a fight for one or two days, then spend some time alone for a few days rethink and reinvest in your values. What core values are important for you in your life? You should take any chance of good communication to resolve the fight. Be honest to yourself about who you are and don't try to pretend to be someone else. Revisit the thoughts with an open mind to see how frequently you're having trouble going through them over a period of time. Be true about your relationship by accepting your mistakes. This will help you to understand what you want or don't want for your future relationship in an honest way. Listen to your gut before making any decision or take more time together to resolve a major issue. If it is not worth wasting your energy on the things you cannot control or you cannot solve yourself first, then ask for outside help. There is no shame in asking for help with marriage counseling to save your marriage. Parents' guidance can help in the same way as a marriage counselor. Sometimes age and maturity can save your relationship automatically.

Unhealthy relationships occur when both are not happy with each other. Sometimes maybe due to busy work schedules, the spouse is not getting attention, or they may be bored with their spouse after years of marriage. It's possible that one partner intentionally wants to hurt the other to prove they are more attractive than him/her and so people can start cheating. Some people are committed to their marriage and keep cheating with their spouse for no reason. After any reason of cheating, some marriages have run their course and are meant to end. No reason to put in any effort for a dead relationship. Just let it go and move forward. Life is too short to stay unhappy in a miserable relationship.

Relationship with family and friends changes after marriage due to many reasons. In the case of a relationship with siblings, no matter what you do with a true heart there will always be something to find problems with. Just do good and move forward. Don't keep any hopes for any type of return otherwise you will be unhappy for the rest of your life. Same with parents, they do a lot with the kids when we are a baby but when parents get older how many of us have returned the favor by doing our duty. There are always a few exceptions in this world.

Long-distance relationships are easy to maintain with less effort by just talking to the partner once in a while. You can visit them when you want without any force. Freedom is flexible with limited restrictions and more personal space.

Short-distance relationships need balance as chances of making mistakes are higher. Don't be too serious, respect others' opinions, speak less and give some space to each other. Letting your spouse go for a guy's night out or shopping night is the mantra for success.

All relationships need trust, care, mutual respect, loyalty, and faith.

- Trust: Is easy to break but it is hard to earn again. If you keep breaking the trust a few times with the partner, then it may be a character issue.

- Care: We are human beings and we all need care. People remember your care the most when you help them during their lower point in life or at crisis time.

- Mutual Respect: Listen to other's opinion with an open mind and say your point without raising your voice. For this, you have to practice active listening during all discussions.

- Loyalty: It needs time to develop an understanding with each other and keep their secrets. Even when your relationship is over with them, avoid speaking negatively about them.

- Faith: It forms over a while in any relationship. You should not break trust of people who have faith in you.

Break up is hard to deal with. Falling out of love is not fun but again sometimes it is natural. It all depends upon person to person how hard it can hit them. It may take years to overcome or sometimes people may die early as they cannot handle the failure. When trust is lost in a relationship, that impacts future decision-making capabilities. Next time with someone new, you may necessarily not feel that excited. You may hold back a little more on what you should share with your partner in the future. It has a significant bearing on future relationships. Bad experiences set the stage for your expectations and behaviors in future relationships. Sometimes it is good that you have learned from it but most of the time bad relationship impacts are not good in life. Sometimes people get so angry and to show their ex, they move quickly to another relationship without much thought. They keep doing the same mistake again and again in their life without learning.

Often people become bitter with age as bad past sticks in their head and they cannot forget the memories which hurt them the most. Sometimes these bad memories impact their health. People with forwarding thinking, don't dwell on the past, are more likely to live a healthier life.

Bad relationships are toxic as they drain you completely. Keep your relationships simple so that you can make good memories in life.

Summary:

- Avoid imposing your opinions on others. Everyone has their mindset based on their own experience in life. Discussions mostly end up with disagreements and fights.

- There is no safe place on this earth for girls. Girls should use their best judgment and if they sense something wrong then don't move forward. Girls or women don't go against your will and if you think someone is abusing you or doesn't understand the meaning of STOP then take immediate action against them so that you don't have to wait and write the story of "Me Too"

- Teach your boys some good manners on how to treat a girl with respect.

- Avoid overhelping in any relationship as you may lose self-respect.

- Few old-fashioned advices to married women that will help them to keep a good relationship with their spouse.

  - Don't get offended by minor things. Just ignore and don't use bad words.

  - Mother nature has given women a superpower to better organize and maintain a good home. Instead of waiting for your spouse to come back from work and help you. You can do home chores so that work will not suffer and ask him to do some other work when you need help. This is a good way to help each other for good understanding.

  - When your husband is arguing then it is better to keep your mouth shut for that moment. Turn around, go to a lonely place, cry a little bit and wash your face. Everything will be fine again. Discuss with him later when things settle down.

  - Treat your in-laws good. Remember one day you will be in the same boat. Be open-minded. Try to keep yourself in their shoes.

- For any type of women abuse, there should be zero tolerance. Pause your relationship and if it is not working, then let it go and move forward.

Financial Freedom

Financial freedom is the biggest success of life, but it's not easy to achieve and comes with a lot of obstructions. In this world, many people dream of becoming a millionaire. Earning money is not easy and becoming financially free is a challenge. You have to give up on the idea of work-life balance. Everything comes with the price of your time in life. In a day we have 24 hours. It all depends upon you where you want to spend your time: either at work or at home. If you spend more hours at work, then chances are you will climb up the ladder or will be successful in your career. But if you decide to spend time with family then you will have a healthy relationship with your spouse and will raise good kids.

For having a balanced life, you need to spend quality time with your spouse and kids to develop understanding, bonding, and teaching them good values. You may also need extra time in life for supporting your aging parents. You need some time for your fitness and hobbies like exercising, gardening, traveling, hiking, and other adventures. Remember you will not get success in all directions and you have to let go of some of your desires. It all depends on your personal choices in which direction you want to grow. You have to sacrifice, compromise, take challenges as an opportunity, and go to an uncomfortable zone to achieve success. Below I have mentioned a few examples of how people manage their time to become financially free.

A friend of mine, who is a good person with a family and a steady job earns a good income. He works for a local company. He has survived a few waves of layoffs. When I asked, do you think about changing your job, he said with two kids it is better to be local and have flexibility at work. "I like what I do," he said in response, "and it's close to home". "I love my schedule, and I like my boss". He has the flexibility to go to work at 10.00 am, come home for lunch, and leave the office around 6 pm each day. Some people are responsible people and manage their work well. They have a comfortable life. But once they lose their job, it's hard to survive. One unfortunate day arrived when my friend didn't survive the next wave of layoffs. Although the company offered severance pay, he had an overwhelming stress of losing his job and his life became upside down. But luckily after a few months, he found another job out of state with a longer commute. He was confused about whether he could take this job or not. Finally, he joined and, in a few months, changed to another local job as he could not handle the commute. They are a good family leading a respectable middle-class life.

On the other hand, there is an example of Dr. Carl and his wife. Both are doctors. It looks good from the outside as to how lavishly they live but the inside story is different. "No pain no gain." When I asked them how they managed their three kids? I got the answer that his wife had to compromise in her career for a few years when the kids were little. When the kids were young Dr. Carl used to work in the night shift while his wife used to work during the day shift. With the help of a full-time nanny, she used to stay with the kids in the evening to cook the food and help the kids with their homework. He used to work over the weekends at another hospital. Their life was not easy as it looked from the outside.

Raising three kids with good values is not easy. Instead of daycare, they had a nanny for their help, which worked well for them. They had to sacrifice a lot of things, face inconveniences, challenges, and discomforts to somehow balance their life. But of course, they have earned good money to live a better life.

Now all three kids of Dr. Carl are doctors too. When I visited them a few years back, I met with their youngest daughter who is an eye surgeon with her two litter kids. She came back from work around 6.00 pm and was on call that week. She got the emergency call at 2.00 am and she went to the hospital, came back at 4.00 am. Again, in the morning, she went to the hospital at 9.00 am. After she came back at 6.00 pm that night her daughter was not feeling good and cried all night. Of course, they have a nanny but still, she had to be up all night with her daughter. I felt she is living a real hard life. She has some choices but looks like she loves her job. In the end, she earns more than a million dollars per year as a doctor but she's leading a very hard life. She is working hard now that will pay off soon for her comfortable life in the future.

I started my career with a moderate income to balance my life. With my permanent job for a few years, I decided to use that time for planning a family and raised two kids. I realized working on the job was not helping much to live a better life. I felt I was going nowhere in my career. Soon after due to some other reason, I decided to leave the job and joined a consulting job.

After becoming a consultant, I went through few layoffs in my career. The day after the layoffs felt like the worst day of my life. But slowly I tried to maintain the normal routine. Sometimes I missed a night of sleep worrying about when I will go back to work again. I kept on trying until I got success finding another job. Sometimes we have to believe in God as he makes a better plan for us. It always took me more than six months to find another job and I used to run out of unemployment benefits. During the consulting job, I was earning good money, but couldn't sustain the job longer due to outsourcing. It is hard to maintain a balance in life when you want to work and don't have a job. I utilized my time in doing the backlog work which was pending on my list for a long time. Keeping a good attitude and following a daily routine helped me a lot to get back to the work again.

While being a stay at home mom, I always learned some new things like:

- Don't buy the things you don't need it. Spend only on necessary things.

- Think twice before you buy as due to limited space at home, you have to throw the old items to replace them with new items.

- Cook food at home to balance out the budget.

This way I did some smart investments during the course of my life. I had to go through several challenges, and compromises to achieve my financial goals. But now it will help me to fund the college expenses for my kid's education, and hopefully, they will be able to graduate from college without a student loan.

When I am at home, I don't like to sit idle. I will always find something to work on and keep myself busy. I am thinking of early retirement so that I will do some volunteering work to help society and people in need.

It is upon the individual on what they pick. I know a few friends who don't want to give up easy life for work, and that is okay. There is nothing wrong with what you want in life as everyone is unique. But then don't complain after looking at your wealthy friends or family members having an extraordinary life after they worked to make their dreams come true. They have worked hard and made the efforts to reach there. Everything in life is associated with a price tag.

The budget is the roadmap to your financial success. Some tips for managing your budget are as follows

- **Start Saving Early:** As soon as you start your first job open a savings account in a bank and start saving whatever you can. Check the bank fees before opening an account. Most banks offer free checking and savings accounts. If they are charging a monthly fee, then ask them about the free checking options or if they can waive monthly fees. Force yourself to contribute to a 401(k) plan to take the advantage of the company match which is free money. If you are self-employed, be sure to contribute the most you can to Traditional or Roth IRAs. Keep doing this and check your accounts every few months. Your goal should be saving whatever you can but live a balanced life in the end.

- **Control Your Spending:** Most people are not sure how much money they are spending. Most of the time, we use the credit card for buying every small thing. Sometimes people are buying the items on sale whether they need them or not. They just buy it as it is cheap. Maybe you will never use that item. So be careful with these sale items you are collecting in a garage or your closet for years and finally giving it away for pennies in a garage sale.

Stop online shopping unless you need it. It may be easy but mostly expensive than buying in the store in a few cases. Don't buy all brand names as it cost much, instead buy generic. Generic makers often spend less on research and development and advertising and pass those cost savings onto consumers. You can use coupons to get additional discounts. Buying in bulk may cost upfront but will save you money in the long run. For expensive items do some research by comparing between different vendors. Every money you save counts in the end. You can control your budget by cutting few additional things like below:

- ○ **Cell phone upgrades and apps**

  Buying the latest smartphone every few years costs money. You may have to enter a new contract at a higher monthly price. New technology has some superior features which you may or may not use it. Every cellphone plan is different. For saving mobile data you can use a WIFI network at home and wherever else it is available. Sometimes apps use data without notifying you. Install less apps on your phone as it does not help you get organized. Some apps may be good, but the question is how many of them do you use. Many of them just waste your time. If apps cost money on a monthly or yearly basis it is better to get rid of them.

- ○ **Buying coffee and dining out**

  Drinking your favorite coffee at a coffee shop may be a good idea in the morning but that costs a lot of money and the other hassle is you have to drive to the coffee shop. You can save a good amount if you can buy a coffee machine at home and enjoy the same coffee every morning.

Dining out occasionally is fine as we all get bored with homemade food. Dining out everyday costs money. As well as outside food is not healthy most of the time. Eating out few times a week will provide a good balance.

- o **Expensive gym memberships**

  Gym membership is good if you are using it. Sometimes people just take the membership and rarely use it. Some people quit after six months or so. Buy one-time good exercise equipment if you have space in your home so that you can use it anytime. You can also use free internet exercise and workout videos.

- o **Landscaping and gardening**

  You can get good outside exercise by mowing your lawn and doing yard work. Another advantage is you can cut as per your convenience when the lawn needs it. Save hundreds or thousands of dollars per season depending upon your lawn.

- **Expensive makeup**

Everyone wants to look good and ends up paying high prices for makeup and other things. Occasionally expensive makeup is good but remember frequent makeup may not be very good for your skin. Makeup is making you beautiful temporarily and may cause skin problems later. For fixing those skin problems you may have to pay big money to the doctors. Apply fewer chemicals on your body so that you will look naturally beautiful and your skin will have time to breathe. Use natural ways to maintain your skin so that you will age gracefully.

- **Salon and spa**

Remember, going to the salon frequently will not make you look beautiful in the long run. Occasionally it is okay but if you cut down by not going for several times a year, it might save you a few thousand dollars per year. Switching from a luxury salon to a basic barbershop is not a bad idea. Start doing some personal grooming at home. Sometimes people may get toenail fungal infection after going to a nail spa as their equipment's is not sterilized after every use. For treating that fungal infection, you may have to pay medical bills to your doctor.

- **Life Insurance**

  It is a personnel choice but, in some cases, there are circumstances where life insurance may not be necessary. If you're young and healthy without dependents or have enough financial assets to pay for your family's care or if your children are already grown up, then you can probably cut this cost.

- **Limit additional expenses**

  - **Membership and subscription services:**

    Buying online is easy but not cheap sometimes. If not tracked properly you may end up paying more. The concept of going to the mall is dying and online businesses are becoming giant due to convenience. We should give some business to small or local businesses for proper wealth distribution. Many people have at least one or more subscriptions they don't use. Some get auto renewed as you don't keep track of them. Getting rid of these can save you money in the long run. You might be wasting your dollars every month on unnecessary subscriptions.

- **Alcohol:**

  It is good to cut costs on alcohol. People spend hundreds to thousands of dollars a year on alcohol. Save money on drinking less and improve your health too.

- **Dry cleaning:**

  Dry cleaning is good sometimes as it is convenient, but it is quite pricey. After you add all the dry-cleaning costs, it is better to buy new clothes than to spend money on your old stuff. You may be bored of wearing them. Another option is that you can wash your laundry by switching your washer to delicate mode. Then iron it using a good iron and ironing board.

- **Wedding:**

  Attending a wedding is a lot of fun in life, but It comes with a price tag. From a new outfit, shoes, and gifts for the newlyweds, to travel and a possible hotel stay. Depending on how many invites you get you might want to pick and choose only those people who are closest to you and hold off on others. Avoid attending the wedding of every invite you get.

- **Live within your means:** It does not matter how much you earn; all that matters is how much you save. Take the necessary steps to pay off your debts. Create a debt payoff plan that works for you. You should save as much as you can. Take the opportunity to max out your retirement plan. Build an emergency fund for at least six months. Pay down your mortgage and save for your kid's college fund if possible.

- **Avoid credit card debt**: Credit card debt is easy to accrue. If you cannot pay in time it is a dangerous game. High-interest credit card debt can kill your budget. To avoid paying a penalty, you have to make the minimum payments, but you will start collecting debt at high interest over a period of time. That will be hard to manage than the monthly payment. If you cannot pay the full credit card amount per month, then don't use a credit card and use the cash option.

- **Buy a home:** It is a good investment to buy a home, but within your range. Purchase a home when you are in your 20s, 30s, or 40s and pay it down. You will have a whole lot of money in the home in terms of equity. For a mortgage at least put 20 percent of the cost of the house as a down payment and make sure you can afford the total monthly cost of the mortgage, insurance, and property tax.

Summary: For financial freedom, you have to get out of your comfort zone for few years and spend your money smartly without wasting it. It does not matter whether you're just saving a dollar. Small amounts add up over time. Unless you are born into a wealthy family, you have to choose which direction you want to go. Either earn a lot of money by working all the time or spending quality time with family and having a balanced life. You will not get success in both the things.

Pandemic 2020

The Pandemic turned 2020 into a historic year. Coronavirus (COVID-19) world crisis has impacted everyone on this earth. During this uncertain time, a lot of things are beyond our control. Fast-moving life has become still. To prevent exposure to the Coronavirus we all have to live in the new world of staying home, washing our hands, wearing masks outside, and keeping a social distance from other people. Keep calm and do your best that you can. No one ever imagined we will have to live our lives in this new way by staying in a lockdown to save ourselves.

The 1918 influenza pandemic is one of the deadliest pandemics in human history. Millions of people died disproportionately of their age in this pandemic. Scientists think that there may have been multiple factors that triggered the last pandemic. Possible reasons could have been the war, severe six-year climate anomaly, or spread of disease through water bodies.

During the current pandemic, the mortality rate of men is more than women. This may be because the immune system of men is weaker than women. I think Coronavirus is the immunity test for all of us. Immunity is linked with your overall health and what you feed to your body. So, it is important to watch what we eat every day for our good health. Immunity fights back against a bacterial or viral infection in our body. As everyone has a different immune system, the Coronavirus effects are different. The medical field was having a hard time finding the correct combination of medicine to treat the patients. Doctors all over the world are working like crazy to deal with this virus. We are grateful to all the frontline heroes and essential workers for putting their own lives at risk to give treatment to the Coronavirus patients. Doctors themselves are overwhelmed because of working in longer shifts for many months.

With all this going on around us, did we self-analyze what happened to so many people around the world during Coronavirus? No jobs due to shut down, increase in suicidal rates, domestic violence, and more. The mental conditions of people are not good. They are emotionally drained with less visibility about the future. Looks like everyone is on the edge because of the constant stress of living life this way. More people are experiencing extreme anxiety, depression, and post-traumatic stress. Few thousands of people are dying every day. Families are losing their loved ones and cannot say the last goodbyes to them. There is such a depressive atmosphere around the world. All these stresses have impacted so many people around the world. This has long-term impacts on our lives, and we are not sure how the next few years will be.

We already have so much stress in our daily lives related to jobs, relationships, health, finances, unexpected changes in life such as the death of a loved one or divorce. This year the pandemic took the stress and uncertainty to another level. These constant stressful situations impact us physically and mentally in unexpected ways. This may extend over a prolonged period which can lead to serious health conditions. High-stress levels break down your nervous system which can weaken the immune system and over time contribute to a broad range of health problems including anxiety, insomnia, headaches, high blood pressure, heart disease, and inflammation.

Our stressful lives may have an impact on our kids as we are always running around to do our daily chores. In general, technology is making our life easy but not making us smart. We spend a lot of time on the screen every day due to many reasons. The fact is that it impacts our minds and forces us to lead an unhealthy lifestyle. We are trying to find shortcuts to lead our lives. Many times, the teenagers and adults are demotivated and withdraw themselves from society, by quitting school. They don't have any technical skills and are unemployed. They are living with their parents and never coming out from their rooms. Parents provide them with food and other stuff in their rooms. They may be passing their day by internet surfing, video gaming, watching television, or by sitting idle and doing nothing. It is a serious concern as it is impacting all of us around the world especially during a pandemic time when kids are spending more screen time. We are in an isolated bubble for more than one year. If humans are withdrawn from society for a long time, they will feel that their living has no meaning or value and will lead a more miserable life with mental illnesses. Mental illness is growing day by day due to an individualistic society with less human interaction. We all need society to grow, learn and live a happy life.

Did we ever realize what mother nature is telling us? After seeing all these for many months can we re-shift our priorities by asking ourselves two questions:

1. Are we happy in our life?

2. Are we leading a healthy lifestyle with less stress in life?

When we look at the trends in the earlier part of the last century, people were living a better life by eating fresh, and organic food. They were happy by spending time with family and socializing with people. Those are the basic needs to live a more wholesome life. Should we change our focus and priorities by taking some breaks and reduce the speed of life to live better? Take some rest or relaxation time in life by spending quality time with family and loved ones and eating healthy to maintain a harmonious life.

For that first and foremost, take care of yourself. If you are healthy then you will provide support to others. A high-stress lifestyle interferes with a human's mental and physical health. It can even become life-threatening. Positive thinking and emotions help boost your immune system, lower blood pressure, and helps extend your life. Use some stress management strategies that can help you move forward productively.

Manage your lifestyle with less stress

- **Relax and recharge yourself:** As the mind influences the rest of your body, recharge yourself by doing activities you like, such as hiking, entertainments, cooking, happy hour, sitting idle at home doing nothing, or whatever else you may like.

  - **Mind:** Keep your mind busy by doing good things like meditation, reading, playing your favorite sport, playing your favorite musical instrument, or listening to your favorite song. Helping others and socializing with people will help you reduce stress and make you feel better.

- **Body:** Take care of your body by eating healthy, drinking enough water, doing regular exercise, and getting enough sleep.

- **Follow a routine:** For maintaining a daily routine you have to develop good habits by following a schedule to do things on time every day. In this way, you will have better time management for your routine. You don't have to stress your mind to follow different schedules every day. Sometimes you can adopt a few changes but changing every day brings stress in life as you have to go through an uncomfortable zone.

- **Get organized:** Long-term planning does not work in life. Better to do monthly planning. Write down the list of work for a month on a paper, calendar planner, or use an app. After making a to-do list, going carefully week by week helps you to reduce last moment stress and you will not forget important stuff that needs to be done during the week. The advantage of this is that you will use your time well and things will not accumulate for the last moment.

If working on a big project, divide it into small parts. Write down the plan in paper or digital form. Do the planning on how you will be doing the small parts month by month so that you will not miss any important steps. Follow your calendar till you finish all the small projects and towards the end look for any remaining items to finish the whole thing. Just divide and conquer.

Arrange and clean up all your closets, garage, and basement in your home and keep the stuff that you need the most. Some things can be kept that you want to preserve as memories or things of emotional value. Clean up everything else that you are not using for more than a few years by either selling or giving it to someone. Your home should have less clutter for it to look spacious and organized. A crowded home with no space brings disorganization and prevents you from thinking clearly.

- **Reassess your priorities and focus on them:** Buy a planner or use an app and write down all your high-priority goals. Have a deadline for each goal and divide it into small tasks on a weekly or monthly basis. Follow up every month where you are with respect to that task. Try to see how you can do better. If needed reassess it for any mistakes, and then correct it. Keep doing this consistently. If at a certain stage you are bored or demotivated, don't lose track. Motivate yourself so that you keep doing it until you finish it.

- **Time management:** Effectively use your time by doing some planning. It does not matter if it is a small project or a big one. Organize your work based on categories, so that you can finish similar items together. For example, going to different stores in the same trip for finishing up things will save time and gas. You may cut some of your screen time and work on your projects over the weekend. Good planning with a deadline helps to work on it optimally with less stress in life. Check your achievements every few months so that you will have a productive year in the end.

- **Avoid unhealthy lifestyle:** Our body is full of chemicals and we are not sure what reaction it performs inside our body. From the outside mostly we all look good but inside, chemicals are playing a different game. Below are some of the ways to follow for a healthy life.

  o The first is to eat fresh and healthy. Eating fresh and healthy is like giving your body premium quality fuel so that your body will stay healthy longer with fewer medical problems. All the illnesses start from the stomach depending on what you feed your body. So, it is important to watch our diet. Due to GMO and non-organic methods, plants are grown to look good from the outside. They focus on selling to the customers, but foods may have so many chemicals to harm the human body from inside. Food and

Drug Administration (FDA) is doing its best but sometimes it is hard to protect us from unknown hazards in food packaging. Some toxic ingredients and materials can potentially affect our bodies. By eating fewer chemicals, we can try to avoid a few harmful things to stay healthy.

- o Second use cooking utensils made of cast iron and stainless steel instead of nonstick pans. Avoiding canned food consumption and reduce the use of plastics in your daily life.

- o The third is to manage your coping mechanisms by not taking help from alcohol, drugs, smoking, or any other type of unhealthy lifestyle. Redirect your energy by developing some hobbies like painting, knitting, cooking, and others. Remember you are responsible for your actions.

- **Avoid negativity:**

  - o Avoid friends or family members who always speak negatively as these negative talks go to your brain. This may have long-term effects on your health. Pick friends wisely as you cannot choose your family members. Mostly school friends are the best as they don't judge you and have less jealousy from your success. Peace of mind is important in life. Stay away from people who disrespect you and don't see your worth. Just move forward and leave it on God to take care of them.

- o Avoid talking negatively about yourself as it spreads fast and comes back to you. Sometimes we bring negativity to ourselves by talking negatively all day. In Indian mythology whatever you keep repeating during the day, sometimes Goddess Saraswati makes that true. So be careful what negative things you keep saying during the day. Maybe you don't want to regret that later in your life.

- o Avoid road rage. You cannot fight a battle with bad people. Your peace of mind is more important than winning a war with them. Let them go first and they will suffer their consequences.

- **Keep faith:** Believe it or not, God exists somewhere. There is some power in this universe. All prayers with true heart are accepted by God sooner or later, no matter where you do your prayer, either at home or at church. If you don't pray, then do meditation. Remember everyone on this earth has to go through hardships and difficulties to reach great heights in the future. Tough time doesn't last, but it makes you stronger for the future. If one door closes, then another door opens. Keep moving in life don't stop. God makes better plans than us.

Indian Herbs for boosting the immune system

Indian herbs (Ayurveda) have the oldest history since the 2nd century BC. It was the foundation laid by the ancient schools of medicine on how to cure yourself using natural ingredients. Indian herbs help to maintain a good metabolism through diet and nutrition for living a long and healthy life.

My mother-in-law in India during COVID times was making Kadha to boost the immune system of the whole family. Kadha is a traditional Indian medicine made up of Indian herbs which help developing immunity with fewer side effects and it has amazing health benefits too.

1. **Recipe for Kadha:**

    Ingredients:

    - **Tulsi leaves (Indian basil)**
    - **Cinnamon**
    - **Black pepper**
    - **Dry ginger and**
    - **Clove**

Procedure: Boil around 2 or 2 1/2 cups of water and add the above ingredients, cook for at least 7 to 10 minutes or until the water reduces by at least half. Stain it and use honey for sweetening. Avoid using sugar. Kadha is the best remedy against fever and sore throat. It is useful to have it fresh.

2. Tea (Chai): Overall tea is good for health but if you can add ginger to it then   it   will prevent you from getting cold and cough.

Procedure: Make tea your way and add fresh ginger to it. Use Honey or maple syrup for sweetening don't use sugar.

3. Turmeric Milk (Golden Milk): Milk is good for health as it has calcium in it and turmeric has a lot of benefits for health.

Procedure: Boil the milk and add a pinch of turmeric to it. If you want, add a pinch of black pepper. Use Honey for sweetening and don't use sugar. Drink warm golden milk at night for better sleep. It also helps during flu to clear up the congestion.

Summary: The new viruses like Zika, Ebola, variants of Coronavirus, and others will be mutating even more in the future and always attacking us. We cannot treat these viruses all the time by taking a vaccination to save ourselves. We should find ways to survive by boosting our immunity which can defend us against different viruses and pathogens.

Seven Secrets For A Happy Life

Happy life has seven secrets to follow without distraction. Life is short and uncertain, so we all have a right to live a contented life.

- Number one is your health. If you don't have good health, you will be unhappy whatever you do. Maintain good health by doing exercise every day, eat healthy and less. Maintain your routine as it affects your health. Eat and sleep on time. Do meditation for at least 10 minutes a day.

- The second is having enough bank balance so that you don't need any help from anyone. You should live a comfortable life and spend on vacations, dining out with friends and family. You can also help your loved ones or anyone else in need.

- The third is good understanding with a life partner or spouse so that you don't have to bang your head against the wall. It destroys your peace of mind and makes you a bad person. It is better to separate than fighting every day and wasting your life in solving issues forever.

- Fourth is own a home. With a rental, you save the headache of maintenance but with your own home, you have your own space to upgrade as per your needs. Plant your garden, trees, and flowers of your choice. See them grow and blossom which gives you happiness inside.

- Fifth is to avoid the people you don't get along with and stop meeting negative people in life. Don't talk to them to waste your time in explaining the same thing again and again as they will never understand and will make you unhappy or uncomfortable. Stop losing your temper and your voice should not get louder on anyone. Whenever a friend or family member has been rude or bad, just move on as a mature person.

- Six is to stop comparing your life with others to avoid unhappiness. Everyone's situation is different, and they pick the option that is good for them.

- Seventh is to spend some time alone every day to think about yourself. How can you improve yourself to live better? Keep learning good things and develop some good habits. Raise your standard. Help others in need, which will give you internal satisfaction.

Balanced Life

A balanced life can be achieved by doing meditation a few hours every day to get inner peace. After doing meditation for around 29 years, I have reached a state where balanced life is the best. This involves simple living and high thinking. It does not matter whether you are successful and rich or not. How satisfied you are in your life matters the most. Live on minimum materialistic needs with some good friends and family members, but of course good food on your plate. For maintaining a balanced life, you have to maintain an equibalance of your mind and body. Be kind to others and don't judge them as you never know from outside what they went through in their life. Helping others in need will give you happiness which you cannot buy using money. Money cannot buy character, happiness, love, satisfaction, and values but you need money to survive on this earth for food, shelter, and clothing. Besides that, you may not need excess money. Cheating and dishonesty catches up to you in life sooner or later. You are responsible for your actions. All we get in the end is our KARMA.

Follow the daily routine of controlling your mind and body for few months to a year before it automatically becomes your habit. Once you develop this habit it will stay with you for a long time unless you push yourself to change it again.

Daily routine for a balanced life

- Drink one glass of water at room temperature without brushing your teeth in the morning.

- You can drink some tea or coffee in the morning but not too much caffeine.

- Listen to calm music like the Gayatri mantra in the morning so that your mind can focus on your daily tasks. Loud music in the morning makes your mind aggressive.

- Do meditation to help you focus on your daily priorities

- Regular exercise of any form is good for us. You can do walking, biking, or yoga during the day. However, new research shows that taking your workout outside could have an even bigger positive impact on your mental health than doing indoor exercises.

- Eat healthy and less. Eat on time and don't skip your meals.

- Spend some time alone every day

In short, you can reach a balanced life by practicing the items listed below:

Think about what you want in life. It is hard to change our personality as it is built-in into our body. Beliefs, values, and assumptions are hard to change as they are built-in with your personality and invisible to others. Artifacts, behaviors, and habits are visible and easy to change. Respect other's beliefs. Life is your mirror image you will get a reflection of what you are. Be an optimist. Have a passion to chase your dream. See challenges as opportunities. Push yourself to follow your dreams and don't give up. Solve problems. Love what you do. It's not all about the money. Do the best you can. Listen more than you talk to become a team player. Follow the right thing even when no one is watching you. Do hard work in your own way. Don't copy others, be yourself. Try new things when you are young. Time is money. Take a risk and don't be afraid of failure. Believe in yourself. Change your attitude to see good in others. Learn from your's and other's mistakes. Don't repeat your mistakes again. Think big and long term. Have a mentor. Be good and kind to others and you will get good in return. Don't cheat on the person who trusts or loves you. Keep your promises. Lying to others means you are lying to yourself. Actions speak much louder than words. Be resourceful and pay attention to the little things. Surround yourself with good and positive people so that you can learn good qualities from them. Keep life simple. Focus on the quality of life. Have confidence and faith. Raise your standard in life and don't compete with cheap people. Prepare for the future. Have a backup plan if things don't work. Add value to your society.

Summary: In the end, a question comes to our mind why the balanced life, and what is the problem with the life I am living now? If you think you are satisfied with the way you are living your life, it is all good. Everyone is unique and has the right to live life in their own way.

Life Conclusions

Everyone is unique and has their own opinion. Sometimes we disagree with others opinion, but don't put down others if their opinion does not match with yours. There is nothing right or wrong. We have to learn how to respect each other's opinions. While spending our time on this earth we can make good and appropriate decisions based on our circumstances and manage our time. Meditation is a way to clean your mind and make your heart beautiful. Whatever good and bad karma we do, we get the results in the end.

The majority of people are confused about their life and do not have the life they want. They are focused on the wrong things. They are spending their energy in the wrong direction either by setting wrong priorities or by having negative people around them. Negative people create bad energy around you. They give you wrong suggestions as they are not successful in their own life. Their negative thoughts doubt your ability to achieve success. Avoid them and move forward. Take the help of meditation to clear your throughs. Write your goals and revisit till you succeed at them

Take care of yourself first by eating healthy. When the sun is out and birds are chirping, get some exercise outside all year round for more fresh air in your lungs. This improves our mood and mental health too. Also spending time in nature is one of the best things we can do to help ourselves feel grounded and improve our happiness. It saves on gym membership too.

We all make mistakes and should learn from them. Don't push your kids too hard that they break in their life and are forced to make bad decisions. Spend time with your kids. Teach them to do the right things, so that when they grow old police don't have to work on them. Guide your kids at every step so that they become good citizens of the nation.

Treat everyone with respect. You will get what you are giving to others. Increase your horizon by thinking big instead of just thinking about yourself, as we live in an individualistic society. Do your duty with your aging parents when they need you so that you will not have regrets later on. Don't be greedy for inheritance money just do good karma and leave the rest on God. Be grateful for what you have in your life rather than complaining about what you don't have.

No generation is better than the other, they are just different. Every age has certain blind spots. A new generation has less patience. It is more aggressive and ready to adopt new things as compared to the older one. The older one is not open to new ideas to change their opinion and habits.

Last but not least we came to earth empty-handed and will go empty-handed one day. We are all renting our bodies, space, and time on earth. By changing our attitude, we can make good memories in life. Don't waste your time on earth and try to do whatever good you can. Don't be greedy. Remember that peace and wealth are the two different sides of the same coin and you won't get both at the same time. Keep doing good karma and it will pay off in some form.

The purpose of writing this book is to share some examples of my life journey which can help you to lead a better life. Hope you will learn new ideas after reading this book and try to change your life for the better.

Some Famous Quotes

"A man is but a product of his thoughts. What he thinks he becomes." - **Mahatma Gandhi**

"Try not to become a man of success but rather to become a man of value." - **Albert Einstein**

"I've failed over and over and over again in my life. And that is why I succeed." - **Michael Jordan**

"Never doubt yourself. Never change who you are. Don't care what people think and just go for it." - **Britney Spears**

"If you set your goals ridiculously high and it's a failure, you will fail above everyone else's success." - **James Cameron**

"The way to get started is to quit talking and begin doing." - **Walt Disney**

"The greatest glory in living lies not in never falling, but in rising every time we fall." - **Nelson Mandela**

"Success is no accident. It is hard work, perseverance, learning, studying, sacrifice and most of all, love of what you are doing or learning to do." - **Pele**

"Your brain is the most important organ in your body, and what happens in it determines what you think and feel, say and do." - **Rick Hanson**

"You could be the world's best garbage man, the world's best model; it don't matter what you do if you're the best." - **Muhammad Ali**

"Don't let yesterday take up too much of today." - **Will Rogers**

"No one can make you feel inferior without your consent." - **Eleanor Roosevelt**

"There is only one happiness in this life, to love and be loved." -**George Sand**

"One child, one teacher, one book and one pen can change the world." - **Malala**

"It's easy to fool the eye but it's hard to fool the heart." - **Al Pacino**

"If you look at what you have in life, you'll always have more. If you look at what you don't have in life, you'll never have enough." -**Oprah Winfrey**

"The ability to influence people without irritating them is the most profitable skill you can learn." - **Napoleon Hill**

"Any time you have an opportunity to make a difference in this world and you don't, then you are wasting your time on Earth." - **Roberto Clementa**

"Man sacrifices his health in order to make money. Then he sacrifices money to recuperate his health." - **Dalai Lama**

"The root of suffering is attachment." - **Buddha**

"Early to bed and early to rise makes a man healthy, wealthy, and wise." - **Benjamin Franklin**

"The best things in life are free. The second best things are very expensive." **- Coco Chanel**

"The only thing that interferes with my learning is my education." **- Albert Einstein**

"Love all, trust a few, do wrong to none." **- William Shakespeare**

"Someone's sitting in the shade today because someone planted a tree a long time ago." **- Warren Buffett**

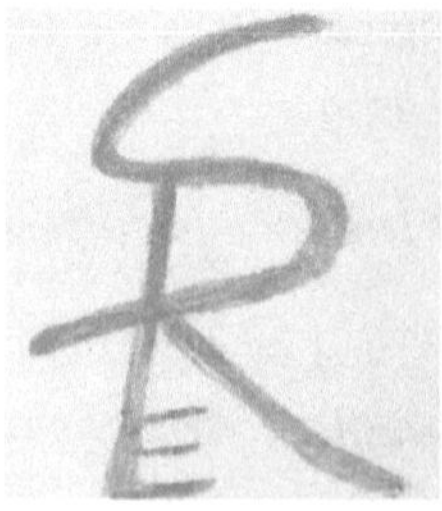